Table Of Contents

Chapter 1: The Benefits of Fitness for Women

Understanding the Importance of Fitness

In today's fast-paced world, it is crucial for women to prioritize their health and overall well-being. Fitness plays a pivotal role in achieving optimal physical and mental health, and it is essential to understand its importance. In this subchapter, we delve into the significance of fitness for women, with a specific focus on high-intensity interval training (HIIT), bodybuilding, and barre workouts for dancers.

Fitness is a gateway to a healthier and more fulfilling life. Regular exercise not only helps in maintaining a healthy weight but also enhances cardiovascular health, boosts metabolism, and strengthens the immune system. Moreover, fitness plays a vital role in managing stress and anxiety, improving mood, and promoting better sleep patterns.

High-intensity interval training (HIIT) has gained immense popularity among women in recent years, and for good reason. HIIT combines short bursts of intense exercises with brief recovery periods, resulting in a highly effective workout that burns calories and boosts metabolism. This form of exercise is time-efficient and can be easily incorporated into a busy lifestyle. By engaging multiple muscle groups and improving cardiovascular endurance, HIIT helps in building strength, increasing energy levels, and enhancing overall fitness.

Bodybuilding is often associated with men, but it holds immense benefits for women as well. Contrary to popular belief, bodybuilding for women does not lead to bulkiness but rather contributes to a sculpted and toned physique. By incorporating resistance training into their fitness routine, women can increase muscle strength, bone density, and metabolism. Furthermore, bodybuilding promotes body confidence and empowers women by challenging societal norms and stereotypes.

For dancers or those interested in graceful and elegant workouts, barre workouts offer a unique and effective approach. Derived from ballet techniques, barre workouts combine elements of dance, Pilates, and yoga to improve flexibility, balance, and core strength. These low-impact exercises target specific muscle groups, leading to long, lean muscles and improved posture. Barre workouts not only enhance physical fitness but also foster a sense of grace and poise.

In conclusion, understanding the importance of fitness is crucial for women seeking to lead a healthy and fulfilling life. Whether through high-intensity interval training (HIIT), bodybuilding, or barre workouts, women can reap numerous benefits, including improved physical strength, enhanced mental well-being, and increased self-confidence. By prioritizing fitness, women can unlock their true potential and achieve a strong and sculpted physique.

The Physical and Mental Benefits of Exercise

In today's fast-paced world, maintaining a healthy body and mind has become more important than ever. Women, in particular, face unique challenges when it comes to fitness. However, with the right knowledge and guidance, women can achieve incredible results and unlock their full potential. This subchapter explores the physical and mental benefits of exercise and how it can transform the lives of women.

Fitness is not just about looking good; it's about feeling strong and confident from within. Regular exercise has been proven to boost self-esteem and improve body image. By engaging in high-intensity interval training (HIIT), women can tap into their inner strength and push their limits. HIIT workouts offer a range of benefits, including increased cardiovascular endurance, improved metabolism, and the ability to burn calories long after the workout is over.

Bodybuilding for women is no longer just a male-dominated domain. With proper guidance, women can sculpt their bodies to perfection and achieve the physique of their dreams. Bodybuilding not only strengthens muscles but also enhances bone density, reduces the risk of osteoporosis, and improves overall body composition. By incorporating weightlifting into their fitness routines, women can develop a lean and toned physique that exudes confidence and power.

For dancers, barre workouts offer a unique blend of strength, flexibility, and grace. Designed to improve posture, strengthen muscles, and enhance flexibility, barre workouts are perfect for women who want to tap into their inner dancer. By combining elements of ballet, yoga, and Pilates, barre workouts sculpt long and lean muscles, improve balance, and boost overall body strength.

Exercise is not just about physical benefits; it also has a profound impact on mental well-being. Regular physical activity releases endorphins, the "feel-good" hormones that combat stress, anxiety, and depression. Women who engage in exercise often report increased energy levels, improved mood, and better sleep patterns. Exercise can also serve as a form of meditation, allowing women to escape the pressures of daily life and find solace in their own bodies.

In conclusion, exercise is a powerful tool that can transform the lives of women. Whether it's through high-intensity interval training, bodybuilding, or barre workouts, women can achieve physical and mental strength that empowers them in all aspects of life. By embracing fitness and making it a priority, women can unlock their true potential and live their lives with confidence, grace, and vitality.

Overcoming Common Obstacles to Fitness

In the journey towards achieving a strong and sculpted physique, every woman encounters obstacles that can hinder progress and motivation. However, with the right mindset and strategies, these obstacles can be overcome, allowing you to reach your fitness goals and unlock your true potential. In this subchapter, we will explore some common obstacles faced by women in their fitness journeys and provide practical solutions to overcome them.

One common obstacle many women face is a lack of time. Between work, family, and other commitments, finding time for fitness can be challenging. However, incorporating high-intensity interval training (HIIT) into your routine can be a game-changer. HIIT workouts are short, intense bursts of exercise that maximize calorie burn and boost metabolism. By dedicating just 20-30 minutes a day to HIIT, you can achieve remarkable results and make the most of your limited time.

Another obstacle that women often encounter is the misconception that bodybuilding is only for men. However, bodybuilding for women is not only possible but also incredibly empowering. By incorporating strength training into your fitness routine, you can build lean muscle mass, increase your metabolism, and achieve a strong and sculpted physique. Embrace the weights and discover the incredible benefits that come with it.

For dancers or those seeking a unique and graceful workout, barre workouts are an excellent choice. However, many women may feel discouraged by the perception that barre workouts are only for professional dancers. Remember, barre workouts are designed to be inclusive and can be modified to suit all fitness levels. By joining a beginner-friendly barre class or following online tutorials, you can develop strength, flexibility, and endurance while enjoying the elegance of dance-inspired movements.

Finally, one of the most significant obstacles women face is the lack of self-confidence. It's essential to remember that every woman's fitness journey is unique, and progress should be celebrated, regardless of how small it may seem. Surround yourself with a supportive community of like-minded women who can inspire and motivate you. Set realistic goals, track your progress, and embrace the process of self-improvement. By cultivating self-confidence, you will see how it translates into every aspect of your life, not just your fitness journey.

In conclusion, overcoming common obstacles to fitness is possible with determination and the right strategies. By making the most of your time, embracing strength training, exploring barre workouts, and cultivating self-confidence, you will be well on your way to achieving a strong and sculpted physique. Remember, you have the power to overcome any obstacle and become the best version of yourself. Let go of limitations and embark on your fitness journey with strength, grace, and unwavering determination.

Setting Realistic Fitness Goals

Setting realistic fitness goals is essential for any woman looking to embark on a fitness journey. Whether you are interested in high-intensity interval training (HIIT), bodybuilding for women, or barre workouts for dancers, understanding how to establish attainable goals is crucial for long-term success.

When it comes to fitness, it's important to remember that progress takes time. Many women fall into the trap of setting unrealistic expectations, only to become discouraged when they don't achieve their desired results overnight. By setting attainable goals, you can create a roadmap to success and maintain motivation throughout your fitness journey.

First and foremost, it's important to establish specific and measurable goals. Instead of saying, "I want to lose weight," set a specific target, such as losing 10 pounds in three months. This allows you to track your progress and adjust your plan accordingly. Additionally, measurable goals provide a sense of accomplishment as you reach each milestone along the way.

Next, it's crucial to set realistic timelines. While we all want to achieve our goals as quickly as possible, it's important to recognize that sustainable change takes time. Rapid weight loss or muscle gain often leads to unsustainable results. Instead, focus on gradual progress that allows your body to adapt and avoids burnout or injury.

Furthermore, it's essential to consider your individual capabilities and limitations. Each woman's body is unique, and what works for one person may not work for another. Be honest with yourself about what you can realistically achieve, both physically and mentally. Setting goals that are too ambitious can lead to frustration and disappointment. Remember, it's about progress, not perfection.

Lastly, seek professional guidance and support. Working with a qualified fitness trainer or coach can help you set realistic goals based on your specific needs and abilities. They can also provide expert advice and keep you accountable throughout your journey. Additionally, surrounding yourself with a supportive community of like-minded women can provide encouragement and motivation along the way.

In conclusion, setting realistic fitness goals is crucial for women in any fitness niche. By establishing specific, measurable goals with realistic timelines and considering individual capabilities, you can create a roadmap to success. Remember, progress takes time, and seeking professional guidance and support can make all the difference. Stay committed, stay motivated, and embrace the journey towards a stronger and sculpted you.

Chapter 2: Introduction to High-Intensity Interval Training (HIIT)

What is HIIT?

HIIT, also known as high-intensity interval training, has gained immense popularity in recent years, particularly among women who are looking to maximize their fitness results in a shorter amount of time. In this subchapter, we will delve into the world of HIIT, exploring its benefits, techniques, and how it can be incorporated into different fitness routines.

HIIT is a form of exercise that involves alternating between short bursts of intense activity and brief recovery periods. These intervals can vary in length, but typically range from 20 seconds to a minute of high-intensity exercise, followed by a rest period of equal or shorter duration. This pattern is repeated for a specific number of rounds, usually lasting around 20-30 minutes in total.

One of the main advantages of HIIT is its ability to increase cardiovascular fitness and burn calories at a much faster rate compared to traditional steady-state cardio workouts. This is because the intense bursts of activity push your body into an anaerobic state, where it relies on stored energy (glycogen) rather than oxygen. As a result, your metabolism is elevated even after the workout, leading to continued calorie burn throughout the day.

Furthermore, HIIT is highly adaptable and can be tailored to suit individual fitness levels and goals. Whether you are a beginner or a seasoned athlete, HIIT can be modified by adjusting the intensity, duration, and rest periods to accommodate your specific needs. This makes it an ideal choice for women who are looking to challenge themselves and push beyond their comfort zones.

Incorporating HIIT into your fitness routine can also complement other forms of exercise such as bodybuilding and barre workouts for dancers. HIIT sessions can be added as a separate workout or integrated into your existing regimen to enhance overall strength, endurance, and flexibility. The explosive movements and quick transitions in HIIT exercises can help build lean muscle, improve coordination, and increase agility, all of which are beneficial for bodybuilding and dance-specific movements.

In conclusion, HIIT is a powerful training method that offers numerous benefits for women in their pursuit of a strong and sculpted physique. Its ability to maximize calorie burn, adaptability to different fitness levels, and compatibility with other exercise modalities make it a valuable addition to any fitness routine. So, whether you're a fitness enthusiast, a bodybuilding enthusiast, or a dancer looking to take your training to the next level, incorporating HIIT into your workouts can help you achieve your goals more efficiently.

How HIIT Benefits Women's Fitness

In recent years, high-intensity interval training (HIIT) has gained immense popularity in the fitness world. This workout methodology involves short bursts of intense exercise followed by periods of rest or low-intensity recovery. While HIIT can be beneficial for both men and women, it offers unique advantages specifically tailored to women's fitness goals. In this subchapter, we will explore how HIIT can help women achieve their desired results, whether it is bodybuilding, overall fitness, or enhancing performance in dance-related activities like barre workouts.

One of the key benefits of HIIT for women is its ability to boost metabolism and burn calories. Research has shown that HIIT workouts can lead to an increased metabolic rate for hours after the session, allowing women to continue burning calories even when they're not exercising. This can be particularly beneficial for women looking to shed excess weight or maintain a healthy body composition.

Moreover, HIIT can help women build lean muscle mass, which is essential for a sculpted and toned physique. Many women fear that weightlifting or intense workouts will make them bulk up, but HIIT provides a balanced approach. By incorporating exercises that target different muscle groups and utilizing bodyweight or light weights, women can achieve the desired muscle definition without excessive bulk.

For women interested in bodybuilding, HIIT can serve as an excellent complementary workout. The short bursts of intense exercise in HIIT sessions can help increase overall stamina, enabling women to perform better during weightlifting or resistance training sessions. Additionally, HIIT can enhance endurance, which is crucial for bodybuilders during competitions or extended training sessions.

Dancers, especially those practicing barre workouts, can also benefit greatly from HIIT. HIIT sessions can improve cardiovascular endurance, allowing dancers to perform better during intense routines. Furthermore, HIIT can enhance muscular strength, flexibility, and coordination, all of which are vital for dancers to execute precise movements and maintain proper form.

In conclusion, HIIT offers numerous advantages for women's fitness. From its ability to boost metabolism and burn calories to helping build lean muscle mass and enhancing performance in various activities, HIIT is a versatile workout regimen that can cater to the specific needs and goals of women. Whether you are aiming to achieve a sculpted physique, improve overall fitness, or excel in dance-related workouts like barre, incorporating HIIT into your routine can be a game-changer in reaching your fitness aspirations.

Safety Considerations for HIIT Workouts

When it comes to fitness, High-Intensity Interval Training (HIIT) has gained immense popularity, especially among women. Its ability to burn fat, increase cardiovascular endurance, and boost overall fitness levels makes it an appealing choice for those looking to get strong and sculpted. However, like any other exercise program, safety should always be a top priority. In this subchapter, we will explore some important safety considerations for HIIT workouts, ensuring that you can enjoy the benefits of this training method while minimizing the risk of injury.

First and foremost, it is crucial to warm up properly before diving into a HIIT session. Performing dynamic stretches, such as arm circles, leg swings, and lunges, helps to increase blood flow, loosen up muscles, and prepare the body for the intense workout ahead. Skipping this step can lead to muscle strains, pulls, or even worse injuries.

Another key safety consideration is to listen to your body. HIIT workouts are intense and push your limits, but it is essential to know when to take a break. Pushing yourself too hard without allowing enough time for recovery can lead to overtraining, fatigue, and even burnout. Remember to pace yourself and gradually increase the intensity of your workouts over time.

Form and technique are also critical when performing HIIT exercises. Proper form ensures that you engage the right muscles and avoid unnecessary strain on your joints. It is advisable to consult a qualified trainer or instructor who can guide you through correct form and provide feedback on your technique to prevent injury.

Furthermore, incorporating rest and recovery days into your training schedule is vital for injury prevention. HIIT workouts put significant stress on your body, and allowing time for recovery allows your muscles to repair and strengthen. Neglecting rest days can lead to overuse injuries and hinder your progress in the long run.

Lastly, if you have any pre-existing medical conditions or injuries, it is essential to consult your healthcare provider before starting a HIIT program. They can provide personalized advice and modifications to ensure your workouts are safe and effective.

In conclusion, HIIT workouts offer tremendous benefits for women looking to improve their fitness levels and achieve a strong and sculpted physique. By following these safety considerations, such as warming up properly, listening to your body, maintaining proper form, incorporating rest and recovery days, and seeking professional advice when needed, you can enjoy the advantages of HIIT while minimizing the risk of injury. Stay committed, stay safe, and enjoy your journey to a fitter, healthier you!

Sample HIIT Workout Routines for Women

High-intensity interval training (HIIT) has gained immense popularity among women due to its effectiveness in burning calories, increasing cardiovascular endurance, and sculpting lean muscles. In this subchapter, we will explore various sample HIIT workout routines specifically designed for women who are seeking to improve their fitness levels, engage in bodybuilding, or enhance their performance in barre workouts for dancers.

1. Fat-Burning HIIT Circuit:
This workout routine is perfect for women looking to shed excess body fat and improve their overall fitness. It involves a combination of bodyweight exercises such as burpees, mountain climbers, jumping jacks, and high knees. Perform each exercise for 30 seconds with maximum effort, followed by a 15-second rest. Repeat the circuit for 4-5 rounds, gradually increasing the intensity as you progress.

2. Muscle-Defining HIIT Workout:
For women interested in bodybuilding, this routine focuses on sculpting and defining muscles. Incorporate exercises like squats, lunges, push-ups, tricep dips, and planks. Perform each exercise for 45 seconds with minimal rest in between. Complete 3 sets of each exercise before moving on to the next. This routine challenges your muscles and helps you achieve a strong and sculpted physique.

3. Barre-inspired HIIT Routine:
Designed especially for dancers or women looking for a low-impact workout with high-intensity benefits, this routine incorporates elements of barre workouts. Include exercises like plié squats, leg lifts, glute bridges, and arm pulses. Perform each exercise for 40 seconds with 20 seconds of rest in between. Repeat the circuit 4-5 times to target specific muscle groups and improve muscular endurance.

It is important to note that before starting any HIIT routine, women should consult with a fitness professional or their healthcare provider, especially if they have any underlying health conditions. Additionally, it is crucial to warm up adequately before each workout and cool down properly afterward to prevent injuries and aid in recovery.

Remember, consistency is key when it comes to achieving your fitness goals. Incorporate these sample HIIT workout routines into your weekly exercise regimen, gradually increasing the intensity and duration as your fitness level improves. Stay committed, push your limits, and enjoy the incredible benefits that HIIT offers.

Chapter 3: Bodybuilding for Women: Building Strength and Confidence

Dispelling Myths about Female Bodybuilding

In today's fitness world, where women are increasingly taking control of their bodies and embracing strength training, there are still many misconceptions surrounding female bodybuilding. These misconceptions often stem from outdated beliefs and stereotypes that need to be debunked. In this subchapter, we will delve into some of the most common myths about female bodybuilding and shed light on why they are far from the truth.

Myth 1: "Lifting weights will make women bulky"

One of the biggest myths about female bodybuilding is the fear of becoming bulky. Many women shy away from weightlifting, thinking they will end up with oversized muscles. However, the truth is that women have lower levels of testosterone compared to men, which makes it extremely challenging to develop bulky muscles naturally. Instead, weightlifting can help women achieve a toned and sculpted physique, enhance metabolism, and improve overall strength.

Myth 2: "Bodybuilding is not suitable for women"

Another common myth is that bodybuilding is a male-dominated sport and not suitable for women. However, this couldn't be further from the truth. Bodybuilding is an inclusive activity that empowers women to build confidence, improve body composition, and enhance overall health. With proper guidance and training, women can participate and excel in bodybuilding competitions, showcasing their hard work and dedication.

Myth 3: "Barre workouts are not effective for building strength"

Barre workouts, often associated with dancers and ballet, are often mistakenly believed to be ineffective for building strength. However, these workouts can be highly effective in toning muscles, improving flexibility, and enhancing overall fitness. Barre workouts combine elements of Pilates, dance, and strength training, creating a unique and challenging exercise routine that targets multiple muscle groups.

Myth 4: "High-intensity interval training (HIIT) is too intense for women"

High-intensity interval training (HIIT) has gained popularity in recent years due to its time-efficient nature and ability to burn calories. However, some women may believe that HIIT is too intense for their fitness level or that it may cause injuries. In reality, HIIT can be tailored to individual fitness levels and provides a variety of modifications to suit different needs. It is an effective way for women to improve cardiovascular endurance, burn fat, and boost metabolism.

By dispelling these myths surrounding female bodybuilding, we hope to encourage women to embrace their strength and pursue their fitness goals without any reservations. Whether you prefer weightlifting, barre workouts, or high-intensity interval training, remember that these activities offer numerous benefits beyond stereotypes, allowing you to achieve the strong and sculpted physique you desire.

Understanding the Benefits of Bodybuilding

Bodybuilding is often misunderstood and wrongly associated with bulging muscles and extreme size. However, for women, bodybuilding offers a plethora of benefits that go beyond just physical appearance. In this subchapter, we will delve into the various advantages of bodybuilding for women and how it can positively impact your fitness journey.

First and foremost, bodybuilding is an excellent form of exercise for overall fitness. It helps to build lean muscle mass, which in turn increases your metabolism, allowing you to burn more calories even at rest. This can be particularly beneficial for women who are looking to lose weight or maintain a healthy body composition. Additionally, bodybuilding enhances strength and endurance, enabling you to perform daily activities more efficiently and reducing the risk of injuries.

Moreover, bodybuilding is an ideal complement to other fitness practices such as high-intensity interval training (HIIT) and barre workouts for dancers. It helps to improve your performance in these activities by increasing your muscular strength and power. By incorporating bodybuilding into your fitness routine, you can take your HIIT sessions or barre workouts to the next level and achieve better results.

Another significant advantage of bodybuilding for women is the positive impact it has on mental well-being. Engaging in regular strength training releases endorphins, commonly known as the "feel-good" hormones, which elevate your mood and reduce stress levels. Furthermore, bodybuilding promotes self-confidence and body positivity, as you witness your body transform and become stronger. This newfound confidence transcends into other aspects of your life, empowering you to overcome challenges and achieve your goals.

In addition to the physical and mental benefits, bodybuilding also contributes to the prevention and management of various health conditions. It helps to increase bone density, reducing the risk of osteoporosis, a common concern for women as they age. Bodybuilding also aids in maintaining healthy blood pressure levels and improving cardiovascular health, reducing the risk of heart diseases.

In conclusion, bodybuilding is a powerful tool for women's fitness. It offers a range of benefits, including increased metabolism, improved strength and endurance, enhanced performance in other fitness practices, boosted mental well-being, and prevention of health conditions. Embrace bodybuilding as a part of your fitness journey, and witness the transformative effects it can have on your body and mind.

Designing an Effective Bodybuilding Program for Women

In the quest for a strong and sculpted physique, women often find themselves in a dilemma. With so much information out there, it can be overwhelming to decide on the right fitness program. This subchapter explores the essentials of designing an effective bodybuilding program tailored specifically for women. Whether you are a fitness enthusiast, a fan of high-intensity interval training (HIIT), a bodybuilding enthusiast, or a dancer looking for barre workouts, this guide is for you.

Strong and Sculpted: A Woman's Guide to Fitness

First and foremost, it is vital to understand that bodybuilding is not just for men. Women can benefit immensely from incorporating bodybuilding exercises into their fitness routine. This program aims to empower women by building strength, enhancing muscle tone, and boosting overall fitness levels.

To design an effective bodybuilding program, it is crucial to set clear goals. Are you looking to improve your overall strength? Or do you want to focus on sculpting specific muscle groups? Once you have defined your goals, tailor your program accordingly. A combination of compound exercises, such as squats and deadlifts, along with isolation exercises, like bicep curls and lateral raises, can help you achieve the desired results.

Additionally, incorporating high-intensity interval training (HIIT) into your bodybuilding program can provide numerous benefits. HIIT workouts are known for their efficiency in burning calories and increasing cardiovascular endurance. Integrate HIIT sessions into your routine to boost fat loss, increase metabolism, and challenge your body in new ways.

For women specifically interested in bodybuilding, it is essential to debunk the myth that lifting heavy weights will make you bulky. In reality, women have lower levels of testosterone, making it difficult to gain significant muscle mass without specific training and dietary protocols. Focus on progressive overload, gradually increasing the weights and intensity of your workouts, to build lean muscle definition and achieve a toned physique.

Lastly, for dancers seeking barre workouts, incorporating elements of ballet-inspired exercises can complement your bodybuilding program. Barre workouts target smaller muscle groups, improve flexibility, and enhance overall body alignment.

Remember, consistency and proper nutrition are key to any successful bodybuilding program. Fuel your body with nutrient-dense foods, stay hydrated, and allow yourself ample time for recovery.

Designing an effective bodybuilding program for women is an empowering journey that can transform your physical and mental well-being. Embrace the challenge, set realistic goals, and watch yourself grow stronger and more sculpted than ever before.

Nutrition Tips for Female Bodybuilders

In the world of fitness, bodybuilding is often associated with men. However, more and more women are stepping into the weight room and embracing the empowering world of bodybuilding. If you are a female bodybuilder or aspiring to become one, it is crucial to understand that nutrition plays a vital role in achieving your goals and maximizing your performance. In this subchapter, we will delve into nutrition tips specifically tailored for female bodybuilders.

1. Prioritize Protein: Protein is the building block of muscle and essential for muscle repair and growth. Aim to consume lean sources of protein such as chicken, fish, tofu, or legumes with every meal. Including a protein shake post-workout can also aid in muscle recovery.

2. Fuel with Complex Carbohydrates: Carbohydrates provide the energy necessary for intense workouts. Opt for complex carbohydrates like whole grains, oats, sweet potatoes, and brown rice. These carbohydrates release energy slowly, keeping you energized throughout your training sessions.

3. Don't Fear Fats: Healthy fats are crucial for hormone production and overall health. Include sources such as avocados, nuts, seeds, and olive oil in your diet. These fats also aid in the absorption of fat-soluble vitamins.

4. Hydration is Key: Staying hydrated is essential for optimal performance. Aim to drink at least eight glasses of water a day. During intense workouts, replenish electrolytes by adding a pinch of salt to your water or opting for natural electrolyte-rich beverages.

5. Adequate Caloric Intake: Female bodybuilders often need to consume more calories to support muscle growth and recovery. Ensure you are eating enough to meet your energy needs and support your training. Consult with a nutritionist to determine your specific caloric requirements.

6. Micronutrient Power: Don't overlook the importance of vitamins and minerals. Incorporate a variety of fruits and vegetables into your diet to ensure you are getting a wide range of micronutrients. Consider adding a multivitamin supplement to cover any potential deficiencies.

Remember, these nutrition tips are specifically aimed at female bodybuilders. Each person's nutritional needs may vary, so it is essential to listen to your body and adjust accordingly. Consulting with a registered dietitian who specializes in sports nutrition can provide personalized advice and help you fine-tune your diet plan.

By prioritizing proper nutrition, female bodybuilders can optimize their performance, enhance muscle growth, and achieve their fitness goals. Embrace the power of nutrition, fuel your body, and witness the incredible transformations that come with a strong and sculpted physique.

Chapter 4: Barre Workouts: Sculpting the Dancer's Body

Exploring the Barre Workout Method

Barre workouts have gained immense popularity in recent years, and for good reason. This unique fitness method combines elements of ballet, Pilates, and yoga to create a low-impact, high-intensity workout that is both challenging and effective. In this subchapter, we will delve into the world of barre workouts, exploring their benefits, techniques, and how they can help women achieve their fitness goals.

One of the main attractions of barre workouts is their ability to sculpt and tone the entire body. By incorporating small, isometric movements, these workouts target specific muscle groups, helping to strengthen and lengthen them. This makes barre workouts an excellent choice for women who are looking to build lean muscle and achieve a sculpted physique.

In addition to strength training, barre workouts also offer a cardiovascular component. The fast-paced, repetitive movements performed in these workouts elevate the heart rate, making them an ideal choice for women who enjoy high-intensity interval training (HIIT). By combining strength and cardio exercises, barre workouts provide a comprehensive full-body workout that helps to burn calories and improve overall fitness levels.

Barre workouts are not only beneficial for women who are new to fitness but also for those with a background in bodybuilding. The controlled movements and focus on form in barre workouts can enhance muscle definition, improve flexibility, and prevent injuries commonly associated with traditional weightlifting. As a result, bodybuilders can supplement their regular training routine with barre workouts to enhance their overall performance and achieve a well-rounded physique.

Furthermore, barre workouts have long been favored by dancers due to their ability to improve balance, coordination, and flexibility. The ballet-inspired movements in these workouts help to strengthen the core, improve posture, and enhance overall body alignment. For women with a background in dance or an interest in barre workouts for dancers, this method can offer a fun and challenging way to stay fit and maintain the grace and poise of a dancer.

In conclusion, barre workouts have become a popular fitness choice for women of all backgrounds and fitness levels. Whether you are new to fitness, a fan of HIIT, a bodybuilder, or a dancer, exploring the barre workout method can bring a plethora of benefits. From sculpting and toning the body to improving cardiovascular fitness, balance, and flexibility, barre workouts offer a comprehensive and enjoyable way to achieve your fitness goals. So grab your mat, put on your ballet flats, and let's dive into the wonderful world of barre workouts.

The Unique Benefits of Barre Workouts for Women

In recent years, barre workouts have gained immense popularity among women of all fitness levels. Combining elements of ballet, Pilates, and yoga, barre workouts provide a unique and effective way to sculpt and strengthen the body. Whether you are a fitness enthusiast, HIIT lover, bodybuilding enthusiast, or even a dancer, barre workouts offer a multitude of benefits that are tailored specifically to women's fitness goals.

One of the most significant benefits of barre workouts is the focus on muscle toning and lengthening. By incorporating small, isometric movements, these workouts target specific muscle groups, such as the thighs, glutes, and core, helping to create long, lean muscles. Unlike traditional strength training exercises that can bulk up the muscles, barre workouts promote a more slender and graceful physique.

Additionally, barre workouts are known for their ability to enhance flexibility and improve posture. The incorporation of ballet-inspired movements helps to elongate the muscles, improving overall flexibility and range of motion. Regular practice of barre exercises can also correct imbalances and alignment issues, leading to better posture and reduced risk of injuries.

For those seeking a high-intensity workout, barre workouts can be modified to meet your needs. By incorporating interval training techniques, such as adding bursts of cardio or incorporating weights, barre workouts can be intensified to challenge even the fittest individuals. This makes it an excellent choice for women who enjoy the intensity of HIIT workouts and want to push their limits.

Barre workouts are also uniquely suited for dancers. As dancers require strength, flexibility, and endurance, barre workouts help dancers improve their technique and overall performance. By focusing on the muscles and movements used in dance, barre workouts can enhance dancers' abilities, allowing them to execute more challenging routines with ease.

Moreover, barre workouts offer a safe and low-impact form of exercise, making them suitable for women of all ages and fitness levels. The low-impact nature of these workouts minimizes stress on the joints while still providing a challenging workout. This makes it an ideal choice for women recovering from injuries or looking for a gentle, yet effective fitness routine.

In conclusion, barre workouts provide a multitude of unique benefits for women in various fitness niches. Whether you are a fitness enthusiast, lover of high-intensity interval training, a bodybuilding enthusiast, or a dancer, barre workouts can help you achieve your fitness goals. From toning and lengthening muscles to improving flexibility and posture, barre workouts offer a holistic approach to women's fitness, resulting in a strong, sculpted, and graceful physique.

Essential Barre Exercises for Strength and Flexibility

In today's fast-paced world, women are constantly seeking ways to stay fit and maintain their health. With the rise of high-intensity interval training (HIIT) and bodybuilding for women, a new fitness trend has emerged that combines the grace of dance with the intensity of strength training – barre workouts. This subchapter will introduce you to essential barre exercises that will help you achieve both strength and flexibility.

Barre workouts have gained popularity among fitness enthusiasts and dancers alike, as they offer a unique blend of ballet-inspired movements and resistance training. These exercises not only sculpt and tone your muscles but also improve your posture and overall body awareness.

One of the most fundamental barre exercises is the plié. Stand with your feet wider than hip-width apart and turn your toes outwards. Slowly bend your knees, ensuring they track in line with your toes. As you rise back up, engage your glutes and inner thighs. Repeat this movement for several reps to strengthen your lower body and improve flexibility in your hips.

Another essential barre exercise is the relevé. Begin by standing with your feet hip-width apart. Rise onto the balls of your feet, lifting your heels off the ground. Squeeze your calves and engage your core as you hold this position for a few seconds. Slowly lower your heels back down to the ground. This exercise targets your calves, ankles, and core, enhancing both strength and balance.

For upper body strength, the push-up is a staple in barre workouts. Start in a high plank position with your hands slightly wider than shoulder-width apart. Lower your body by bending your elbows, keeping them close to your sides. Push back up to the starting position, engaging your chest, shoulders, and triceps. If needed, modify this exercise by performing it on your knees. Aim for a straight line from your head to your knees or toes.

Incorporating these essential barre exercises into your fitness routine will help you build strength, increase flexibility, and improve your overall fitness level. Whether you are a dancer looking to enhance your performance or someone simply seeking a fun and effective workout, barre exercises offer a wide range of benefits for women of all fitness levels. So, grab your sticky socks, find a barre, and get ready to sculpt and strengthen your body like never before.

Incorporating Barre Workouts into Your Fitness Routine

Barre workouts have gained tremendous popularity in recent years, and for good reason. This unique exercise method combines elements of ballet, Pilates, and yoga to create a challenging yet graceful workout that targets multiple muscle groups. Whether you're a fitness enthusiast, a dancer, or simply looking to add variety to your exercise routine, incorporating barre workouts can provide numerous benefits for your body and mind.

For women looking to achieve a lean and sculpted physique, barre workouts offer a perfect solution. By utilizing isometric movements and small, controlled pulses, these workouts effectively tone and strengthen muscles without adding bulk. This is particularly appealing to women who want to maintain a feminine shape while building strength and endurance. Furthermore, barre workouts focus on the core, legs, and glutes, areas that are often a priority for women seeking a well-balanced physique.

If you're a fan of high-intensity interval training (HIIT), you'll be pleasantly surprised by the intensity of a barre workout. While the movements may appear graceful and fluid, they require immense strength and endurance. The combination of repetitive exercises and targeted muscle engagement creates an intense burn that boosts your heart rate and torches calories. By incorporating barre workouts into your fitness routine, you'll be able to enjoy the benefits of both strength training and cardiovascular exercise.

Bodybuilding for women is no longer limited to lifting heavy weights. Barre workouts provide an excellent complement to traditional weightlifting routines. By incorporating barre exercises into your strength training program, you can enhance your muscle definition, improve flexibility, and prevent injuries. The isometric holds and controlled movements in barre workouts help to strengthen the stabilizing muscles, which are often neglected in traditional bodybuilding workouts.

Lastly, if you're a dancer looking to improve your technique or recover from an injury, barre workouts are an excellent addition to your training regimen. These workouts focus on alignment, flexibility, and balance, all of which are crucial for dancers to perform at their best. Barre workouts can help dancers build strength in their supporting muscles, increase flexibility in their hips and legs, and improve their overall body awareness.

Incorporating barre workouts into your fitness routine can provide a wealth of benefits, regardless of your fitness goals. Whether you're looking to tone and sculpt your body, boost your cardiovascular fitness, enhance your strength training, or improve your dance performance, barre workouts offer a versatile and effective solution. So, grab your ballet slippers, embrace your inner dancer, and get ready to experience the transformative power of barre workouts.

Chapter 5: Nutrition and Meal Planning for Women's Fitness

The Role of Nutrition in Women's Fitness

Nutrition plays a crucial role in women's fitness, supporting overall health and enhancing performance in various fitness activities such as high-intensity interval training (HIIT), bodybuilding, and barre workouts for dancers. In this subchapter, we will delve into the importance of proper nutrition for women and how it can optimize their fitness journey.

First and foremost, it is essential to understand that women's nutritional needs differ from those of men due to various physiological factors. A well-balanced diet that includes an adequate amount of macronutrients, such as proteins, carbohydrates, and healthy fats, is vital for women engaging in fitness activities. These macronutrients provide the necessary fuel for energy, muscle recovery, and growth.

High-intensity interval training (HIIT), a popular form of exercise among women, demands a significant amount of energy. To support HIIT workouts, women should focus on consuming complex carbohydrates like whole grains, fruits, and vegetables, as these provide sustained energy throughout the session. Additionally, lean proteins such as chicken, fish, tofu, and legumes are essential for muscle repair and growth. Including healthy fats from sources like avocados, nuts, and olive oil can aid in hormone production and overall health.

For women interested in bodybuilding, nutrition becomes even more critical. Building lean muscle mass requires a higher intake of protein to repair and develop muscles. Protein sources like lean meats, eggs, dairy products, and plant-based proteins such as quinoa and lentils should be a part of daily meals. Adequate hydration is also vital for muscle recovery and overall performance, so drinking enough water throughout the day is crucial.

Barre workouts are a unique fitness activity for dancers and women seeking a low-impact yet challenging exercise routine. Proper nutrition is vital in supporting endurance and flexibility necessary for barre workouts. Including a variety of fruits, vegetables, whole grains, and lean proteins in one's diet can aid in maintaining a healthy weight and providing sustained energy during these workouts.

In conclusion, nutrition plays a pivotal role in women's fitness, regardless of the chosen niche such as high-intensity interval training (HIIT), bodybuilding, or barre workouts for dancers. A well-balanced diet that includes macronutrients like proteins, carbohydrates, and healthy fats is essential for providing energy, supporting muscle growth and recovery, and optimizing overall performance. By prioritizing nutrition alongside regular exercise, women can achieve their fitness goals, improve their overall health, and lead a strong and sculpted life.

Understanding Macronutrients and Micronutrients

In the world of fitness, it is crucial for women to have a solid understanding of macronutrients and micronutrients. These two categories of nutrients play a vital role in fueling your workouts, aiding in muscle recovery and growth, and maintaining overall health and well-being. Whether you are engaged in high-intensity interval training (HIIT), bodybuilding, or barre workouts for dancers, knowing how to properly nourish your body can make a significant difference in achieving your fitness goals.

Macronutrients are the nutrients that our bodies require in large quantities. They include carbohydrates, proteins, and fats. Carbohydrates are the primary source of energy for our bodies, and they are especially important for high-intensity workouts. Incorporating complex carbohydrates such as whole grains, fruits, and vegetables into your diet will provide sustained energy and prevent fatigue during your workouts. Proteins are essential for muscle repair and growth. Including lean sources of protein like chicken, fish, tofu, or Greek yogurt in your meals will aid in recovery and promote muscle development. Healthy fats, such as avocados, nuts, and olive oil, are essential for hormone production and cell maintenance.

On the other hand, micronutrients are the nutrients that our bodies require in smaller quantities but are equally essential for optimal health. These include vitamins and minerals. Vitamins, such as vitamin C, B vitamins, and vitamin D, play a crucial role in energy production, immune function, and bone health. Minerals, such as calcium, iron, and magnesium, are important for muscle contraction, oxygen transport, and maintaining electrolyte balance. Consuming a variety of colorful fruits and vegetables, whole grains, lean proteins, and dairy products will ensure you are getting an array of essential micronutrients.

Understanding the balance between macronutrients and micronutrients is key to achieving your fitness goals. While macronutrients provide the energy and building blocks, micronutrients support overall health and ensure your body functions optimally. A well-balanced diet that includes a variety of nutrient-dense foods will help you achieve optimal performance, enhance recovery, and promote overall well-being.

It is essential to note that individual nutritional needs may vary based on factors such as age, activity level, and specific fitness goals. Consulting with a registered dietitian or nutritionist can provide personalized guidance and help you create a nutrition plan tailored to your unique needs. By nourishing your body with the right balance of macronutrients and micronutrients, you can maximize your fitness journey and achieve a strong and sculpted physique.

Creating a Balanced Meal Plan for Optimal Fitness

Nutrition plays a crucial role in achieving optimal fitness. As women, we have unique needs when it comes to fueling our bodies for high-intensity interval training (HIIT), bodybuilding, or barre workouts. To support our active lifestyles and sculpted physiques, it's important to create a balanced meal plan that provides all the necessary nutrients. Let's dive into the essential components of a well-rounded diet for women in the fitness niche.

Protein, the building block of muscle, should be a key focus in our meal plan. Whether we are engaging in HIIT, bodybuilding, or barre workouts, protein is essential for muscle repair and growth. Include lean sources of protein in each meal such as chicken, turkey, fish, tofu, or legumes. Aim for a serving size of around 20-30 grams per meal to maximize muscle recovery and development.

To support our energy levels and overall health, we need to incorporate complex carbohydrates into our meal plan. These include whole grains, brown rice, quinoa, and sweet potatoes. Complex carbs provide sustained energy, helping us power through intense workouts and maintain optimal performance.

Healthy fats are another vital component of our meal plan. Avocados, nuts, seeds, and olive oil are excellent sources of healthy fats that provide essential nutrients and aid in hormone balance. Including these fats in our diet can improve our body's ability to absorb fat-soluble vitamins and promote a healthy brain function.

Vitamins and minerals are essential for overall wellness. Women often have specific nutrient needs, such as iron and calcium. Leafy greens, lean red meat, and fortified cereals are excellent sources of iron, while dairy, tofu, and leafy greens provide calcium. Be sure to incorporate a variety of fruits and vegetables to ensure you're getting a wide range of essential vitamins and minerals.

Hydration is key for optimal fitness. Drinking enough water throughout the day not only keeps us hydrated but also aids in digestion and nutrient absorption. Aim to drink at least eight cups of water daily, and consider adding electrolyte-rich beverages to replenish minerals lost during intense workouts.

In conclusion, creating a balanced meal plan is essential for women in the fitness niche. By incorporating lean protein, complex carbohydrates, healthy fats, vitamins, minerals, and staying hydrated, we can support our bodies in achieving optimal fitness, whether we're engaged in HIIT, bodybuilding, or barre workouts. Remember, a well-nourished body is a strong and sculpted body.

Tips for Healthy Eating on a Busy Schedule

In today's fast-paced world, it can be challenging for women to maintain a healthy diet while juggling various responsibilities. However, with a little planning and some smart choices, it is possible to make nutritious eating a priority even on a busy schedule. Here are some valuable tips to help you achieve a healthy diet and optimal fitness levels while managing your everyday tasks.

1. Plan Your Meals in Advance: Take a few minutes each week to plan your meals ahead. This will save you time and ensure you have nutritious options readily available. Consider batch cooking and meal prepping on weekends to have healthy meals and snacks ready to grab during the busy workweek.

2. Keep Healthy Snacks Handy: Stock your pantry and desk drawer with nutritious snacks like nuts, seeds, dried fruits, or protein bars. These options will provide sustained energy and keep you away from unhealthy vending machine temptations.

3. Prioritize Protein: Protein is essential for muscle recovery and growth, making it a crucial component of any fitness routine. Include lean sources of protein like chicken, fish, tofu, or legumes in your meals to support your workouts and promote muscle development.

4. Embrace Quick and Easy Recipes: Look for recipes that are both healthy and time-efficient. Opt for meals that can be prepared in under 30 minutes, such as stir-fries, salads, or sheet pan dinners. Utilize time-saving kitchen tools like slow cookers or instant pots to make cooking a breeze.

5. Opt for Whole Foods: Choose whole, unprocessed foods whenever possible. These foods are packed with essential nutrients and are less likely to contain added sugars, unhealthy fats, or artificial additives. Incorporate plenty of fruits, vegetables, whole grains, and lean proteins into your diet.

6. Stay Hydrated: Proper hydration is crucial for overall health and fitness. Keep a water bottle with you at all times and aim to drink at least eight glasses of water per day. If plain water gets monotonous, infuse it with natural flavors like lemon, cucumber, or mint.

7. Be Mindful of Portion Sizes: Even with healthy choices, overeating can still hinder your progress. Pay attention to portion sizes and listen to your body's hunger and fullness cues. Avoid eating in front of screens, as it can lead to mindless overeating.

Remember, healthy eating is not about depriving yourself but rather nourishing your body to perform at its best. By incorporating these tips into your daily routine, you can maintain a balanced diet and achieve your fitness goals, even with a busy schedule.

Chapter 6: Injury Prevention and Recovery for Women

Common Injuries in Women's Fitness

As women, we strive to achieve our fitness goals and maintain a healthy lifestyle. Whether you're into high-intensity interval training (HIIT), bodybuilding, or barre workouts for dancers, it's important to be aware of the common injuries that can occur during these activities. By understanding these potential risks, you can take precautions and make informed choices to prevent injury and continue on your fitness journey.

One common injury in women's fitness is sprains and strains. These can occur when we push ourselves too hard or don't warm up properly before a workout. HIIT workouts, with their intense bursts of activity, can put excessive strain on our muscles and joints if not performed with proper technique. Similarly, bodybuilding exercises that involve heavy weights can lead to strains if we lift more than our bodies can handle. To avoid these injuries, it's crucial to warm up before each workout, stretch properly, and listen to your body's limits.

Another common injury is tendonitis, which is the inflammation of a tendon. This can happen when we repeatedly perform the same movements, such as those found in bodybuilding or barre workouts. Tendonitis often affects areas like the shoulders, wrists, and ankles. Taking breaks between workouts, using proper form, and incorporating exercises that target different muscle groups can help prevent tendonitis.

Knee injuries are also prevalent in women's fitness, especially in activities that involve jumping or repetitive knee movements, like HIIT and barre workouts. Conditions such as runner's knee or patellar tendonitis can develop if the knees are not properly supported or if there is an imbalance in the muscles surrounding the knee joint. Wearing supportive footwear, using knee braces if necessary, and incorporating exercises that strengthen the quadriceps and hamstrings can help protect the knees from injury.

Lastly, back injuries are a concern for women engaged in bodybuilding exercises, especially if proper form and technique are not followed. Deadlifts, squats, and other compound movements can strain the back if the core muscles are not engaged or if we lift weights that are too heavy. It's crucial to start with lighter weights, focus on proper form, and gradually increase the load to avoid back injuries.

In conclusion, being aware of the common injuries that can occur in women's fitness is essential for maintaining a safe and effective workout routine. By warming up, using proper form, incorporating variety in your exercises, and listening to your body, you can reduce the risk of sprains, strains, tendonitis, knee injuries, and back problems. Remember, the goal is not just to get fit but also to remain strong and sculpted for the long term.

Prehabilitation Exercises for Injury Prevention

In the pursuit of a strong and sculpted physique, it is essential for women to prioritize injury prevention. To ensure a long and successful fitness journey, incorporating prehabilitation exercises into your routine is crucial. Prehabilitation refers to exercises and techniques that proactively address potential imbalances, weaknesses, and limitations in the body, reducing the risk of injury. By taking proactive steps, you can safeguard yourself against the setbacks that injuries can cause, allowing you to stay consistent and progress towards your fitness goals.

One effective method to prevent injuries is by incorporating high-intensity interval training (HIIT) into your fitness routine. HIIT workouts are known for their efficiency and effectiveness, but they can also put stress on the body if not properly prepared. Engaging in dynamic warm-up exercises, such as leg swings, arm circles, and torso rotations, helps activate and prepare the muscles, tendons, and joints for the demands of a HIIT session. This warm-up routine enhances flexibility, increases blood flow, and improves range of motion, reducing the risk of strains and sprains.

Bodybuilding for women has gained significant popularity in recent years, and with it comes the importance of injury prevention. Focusing on compound exercises like squats, deadlifts, and bench presses can lead to tremendous gains in strength and muscle mass. However, these exercises also place substantial stress on the body. Incorporating prehabilitation exercises, such as glute bridges, clamshells, and lateral band walks, can help activate and strengthen the muscles surrounding the hips, knees, and ankles. Stronger stabilizing muscles reduce the risk of joint injuries and improve overall performance in the gym.

Barre workouts, designed to mimic the movements of ballet dancers, are excellent for building strength, flexibility, and grace. However, the repetitive nature of these workouts can lead to overuse injuries if certain precautions are not taken. Incorporating exercises that target the feet and ankles, such as calf raises, ankle circles, and toe scrunches, can improve stability and mobility in these areas. Additionally, focusing on core stability exercises, like planks and side planks, can enhance overall balance and reduce the risk of falls or strains during barre workouts.

Prehabilitation exercises for injury prevention should be an integral part of every woman's fitness routine. By taking proactive measures to address potential imbalances and weaknesses, you can stay injury-free and continue progressing towards your goals. Remember, prevention is always better than cure, and by incorporating these exercises, you can have a solid foundation for a strong, sculpted, and injury-free body.

Rehabilitation Strategies for Common Fitness Injuries

In the pursuit of a strong and sculpted body, women often push themselves to their limits during fitness activities such as high-intensity interval training (HIIT), bodybuilding, and barre workouts for dancers. While these workouts can be incredibly effective in achieving fitness goals, they also come with the potential risk of injuries. It is essential for women to be aware of common fitness injuries and have a solid understanding of rehabilitation strategies to promote a safe and effective recovery.

One of the most common fitness injuries is muscle strain. This occurs when the muscle fibers are stretched or torn due to overexertion or improper form during exercises. To rehabilitate a strained muscle, it is crucial to follow the RICE (rest, ice, compression, elevation) method. Resting the injured muscle allows it to heal, while applying ice and compression reduces swelling and pain. Elevation helps to drain excess fluid from the injured area. Additionally, gentle stretching and strengthening exercises under the guidance of a professional can aid in the recovery process.

Another frequent injury among fitness enthusiasts is tendonitis, which is the inflammation of a tendon. This can be caused by repetitive movements or poor technique during exercises. To rehabilitate tendonitis, it is important to rest the affected area and avoid activities that aggravate the condition. Applying heat or ice, performing stretching exercises, and using supportive braces or wraps can also provide relief. Gradually reintroducing exercises and activities, with a focus on proper form and technique, can help prevent reinjury.

Stress fractures are another injury that can result from high-impact activities or excessive training. These tiny cracks in the bone require a longer recovery period. Rest is crucial for healing stress fractures, along with the use of crutches or a walking boot to reduce weight-bearing. Low-impact exercises like swimming or cycling can be incorporated during the recovery process to maintain cardiovascular fitness.

Injuries in the fitness world are not uncommon, but they shouldn't deter women from pursuing their fitness goals. By understanding common fitness injuries and the appropriate rehabilitation strategies, women can take proactive measures to prevent and recover from injuries effectively. Remember, consulting with a healthcare professional or a qualified trainer is always recommended to ensure proper diagnosis and personalized guidance throughout the rehabilitation process. With the right approach, women can safely and confidently continue their fitness journeys, achieving strength and sculpted bodies while prioritizing their overall well-being.

Listening to Your Body: Rest and Recovery

In our modern, fast-paced world, it's easy to get caught up in the hustle and bustle of daily life. As women, we often juggle multiple responsibilities, leaving little time for ourselves. However, it's crucial to prioritize rest and recovery in our fitness journey. In this subchapter, we will delve into the importance of listening to your body and how rest and recovery contribute to achieving a strong and sculpted physique.

Fitness is not just about pushing your limits; it's also about knowing when to give your body a break. High-intensity interval training (HIIT), bodybuilding, and barre workouts for dancers all require immense physical exertion. While these activities can be exhilarating and empowering, they also put strain on our muscles and joints. Ignoring the signs of fatigue and overtraining can lead to injuries and setbacks.

Listening to your body means paying attention to its signals. If you feel excessively sore, fatigued, or experience decreased performance, it's your body's way of telling you it needs rest. Rest days are not a sign of weakness, but rather an essential component of any fitness regimen. They allow your body to repair and rebuild itself, leading to improved strength and endurance.

Recovery is just as important as rest. Proper nutrition, hydration, and sleep are vital for the body to recharge and replenish. Adequate protein intake is especially crucial for women engaged in bodybuilding or intense workouts. Protein aids in muscle repair and growth, ensuring you achieve the sculpted physique you desire. Hydration is vital for maintaining optimal performance and preventing muscle cramps, while quality sleep promotes hormone regulation and muscle recovery.

Additionally, active recovery techniques can enhance your overall fitness journey. Incorporating activities like yoga, stretching, or low-intensity cardio on rest days can improve flexibility, reduce muscle soreness, and increase blood flow to aid in recovery.

Remember, every woman's body is unique, and what works for one may not work for another. It's essential to listen to your body's individual needs and adjust your fitness routine accordingly. By incorporating rest and recovery into your fitness journey, you will not only prevent burnout and injuries but also achieve your fitness goals more effectively.

In conclusion, listening to your body and prioritizing rest and recovery is crucial for women in the world of fitness. Whether you engage in high-intensity interval training, bodybuilding, or barre workouts for dancers, taking the time to rest and recover will lead to a stronger, sculpted physique. Embrace rest days, fuel your body with proper nutrition, and practice active recovery techniques to optimize your fitness journey. Remember, self-care is not selfish; it's an essential part of achieving your fitness goals and maintaining overall well-being.

Chapter 7: Motivation and Mental Well-being for Women's Fitness

Staying Motivated on Your Fitness Journey

Introduction:
Embarking on a fitness journey can be an exciting and empowering endeavor for women. Whether you are interested in high-intensity interval training (HIIT), bodybuilding, or barre workouts for dancers, maintaining motivation is key to achieving your fitness goals. In this subchapter, we will explore effective strategies and techniques to help you stay motivated on your fitness journey, ensuring that you reach new heights and sculpt the strong, confident body you desire.

Setting Clear Goals:
To stay motivated, it is crucial to establish clear and realistic goals. Determine what you want to achieve, whether it is boosting your endurance, building muscle, or perfecting your dance moves. Write down your goals and break them into smaller, achievable milestones. Celebrate your progress along the way, as each accomplishment will fuel your motivation further.

Tracking Progress:
Tracking your progress is a powerful tool to stay motivated. Keep a record of your workouts, noting the exercises, sets, and repetitions completed. Additionally, take regular measurements and photos of your body to track changes in strength, muscle definition, and overall physique. Seeing tangible evidence of your progress will inspire you to keep pushing forward.

Finding Support:
Surrounding yourself with a supportive community is essential for staying motivated. Seek out like-minded individuals who share your fitness goals and interests. Join fitness classes, online forums, or local fitness groups where you can connect with other women who are on a similar journey. Sharing experiences, providing encouragement, and receiving support from others will keep you motivated during challenging times.

Varying Your Workouts:
Monotony can quickly drain your motivation. Keep your workouts fresh and exciting by incorporating a variety of exercises and training methods. If you enjoy HIIT workouts, try different interval patterns or experiment with new exercises to keep your routine dynamic. If bodybuilding is your focus, switch up your exercises, incorporate different rep ranges, or try new lifting techniques. For barre workouts, explore different styles and techniques to challenge your body and mind. By continually introducing new elements to your workouts, you will stay engaged and motivated to push your limits.

Rewarding Yourself:
Rewarding yourself along the way is vital to maintain motivation. Set up a system of rewards for reaching your fitness milestones, such as treating yourself to a massage, buying new workout gear, or indulging in a guilt-free cheat meal. These rewards will serve as positive reinforcement and give you something to look forward to as you progress on your fitness journey.

Conclusion:
Staying motivated on your fitness journey is crucial for achieving your goals in fitness, whether it's through HIIT, bodybuilding, or barre workouts. By setting clear goals, tracking your progress, finding support, varying your workouts, and rewarding yourself, you will maintain the motivation necessary to sculpt a strong and confident body. Remember, motivation is not always constant, but with the right strategies in place, you can overcome obstacles and continue striving towards your fitness aspirations. Stay focused, stay motivated, and embrace the incredible transformation that awaits you.

Overcoming Mental Barriers to Fitness Success

Introduction:
In the journey to achieving a strong and sculpted physique, women often encounter mental barriers that hinder their progress. These barriers can range from self-doubt and lack of motivation to fear of failure or judgment. However, it is important to recognize that these barriers are not insurmountable. By understanding and addressing them head-on, women can overcome their mental obstacles and unlock their true fitness potential. In this subchapter, we will explore various strategies and techniques to conquer these mental barriers and pave the way for fitness success.

1. Self-Doubt:
One of the most common mental barriers faced by women is self-doubt. Many women doubt their abilities, compare themselves to others, or believe they are not strong or capable enough. To overcome self-doubt, it is crucial to develop a positive mindset and focus on personal progress rather than external comparisons. Setting achievable goals, celebrating small victories, and surrounding oneself with a supportive community can also help build confidence and overcome self-doubt.

2. Lack of Motivation:
Maintaining consistent motivation can be challenging, especially when faced with busy schedules or fatigue. To overcome this mental barrier, it is essential to find intrinsic motivations that resonate with individual passions and values. Creating a workout routine that includes enjoyable activities, finding an exercise buddy, or seeking professional guidance can reignite motivation and make fitness a sustainable habit.

3. Fear of Failure:
Fear of failure can hinder women from pushing their limits and taking risks in their fitness journey. To overcome this fear, it is crucial to reframe failure as an opportunity for growth and learning. Embracing a growth mindset, setting realistic expectations, and viewing setbacks as stepping stones rather than roadblocks can empower women to embrace challenges and conquer their fears.

4. Fear of Judgment:
The fear of judgment can often prevent women from fully committing to their fitness goals. However, it is important to remember that everyone has their own journey and struggles. Surrounding oneself with a non-judgmental and supportive community, practicing self-compassion, and focusing on personal progress rather than external opinions can help overcome this mental barrier.

Conclusion:
In conclusion, overcoming mental barriers is a crucial aspect of achieving fitness success for women. By recognizing and addressing self-doubt, lack of motivation, fear of failure, and fear of judgment, women can break free from these mental barriers and unlock their full fitness potential. Through cultivating a positive mindset, setting achievable goals, seeking support, and embracing challenges, women can pave the way to a strong and sculpted physique. Remember, your mental strength is just as important as your physical strength on the journey to fitness success.

Incorporating Mindfulness and Self-Care into Your Routine

In today's fast-paced and demanding world, it's crucial for women to prioritize their overall well-being, both physically and mentally. While focusing on fitness goals like high-intensity interval training (HIIT), bodybuilding, or barre workouts, it's equally important to integrate mindfulness and self-care practices into your routine. By doing so, you can achieve a harmonious balance between pushing your limits and nurturing your mind and body.

Mindfulness, often associated with meditation, is a practice that cultivates present-moment awareness and promotes a deeper connection with ourselves. As women, we tend to juggle numerous responsibilities, whether it's work, family, or personal goals. Incorporating mindfulness into your fitness routine allows you to be fully present during your workouts, enhancing the mind-body connection and maximizing the benefits of your efforts.

Begin by setting aside a few minutes each day for mindfulness exercises. Find a quiet space, close your eyes, and focus on your breath. Notice the sensations in your body and let go of any thoughts or distractions. This simple act of mindfulness can help reduce stress, increase concentration, and improve your overall mental well-being.

Self-care is another essential element to integrate into your routine. As women, we often put others' needs before our own, neglecting our own self-care. However, taking care of ourselves is crucial for maintaining physical and mental health. Prioritize activities that bring you joy and help you relax, such as taking a long bath, reading a book, or practicing hobbies outside of fitness. Remember, self-care is not selfish; it is necessary for self-preservation.

Another aspect of self-care is ensuring you provide your body with the necessary recovery and rest. Your muscles need time to repair and grow after intense workouts. Adequate sleep, proper nutrition, and listening to your body's cues for rest are vital components of self-care. Neglecting these aspects can lead to burnout, injuries, and hinder your progress towards your fitness goals.

Incorporating mindfulness and self-care practices into your routine can transform your fitness journey. By nurturing your mind and body, you'll find increased motivation, mental clarity, and a heightened sense of well-being. Remember, fitness is not just about physical strength; it's also about achieving a balanced and fulfilled life. Embrace mindfulness and self-care to become strong and sculpted from the inside out.

Celebrating Your Achievements and Maintaining Long-Term Fitness

As women, we often strive to achieve our fitness goals, whether it's improving our strength, sculpting our bodies, or excelling in a specific workout niche. In this subchapter, we will explore the importance of celebrating your achievements and provide guidance on maintaining long-term fitness success.

Fitness is not just about physical transformation; it's also about recognizing and celebrating the milestones you've achieved along the way. Take a moment to acknowledge your progress, whether it's hitting a personal best in a high-intensity interval training (HIIT) workout or successfully completing a challenging barre routine. Celebrating these achievements boosts your confidence, motivates you to keep going, and reinforces your commitment to your fitness journey.

To maintain long-term fitness, it's crucial to establish sustainable habits that support your goals. One effective approach is incorporating a variety of workout styles into your routine. High-intensity interval training (HIIT) is an excellent option for women looking to maximize their fitness gains in a short amount of time. HIIT workouts challenge your cardiovascular system while engaging multiple muscle groups, resulting in increased calorie burn and improved overall fitness levels.

For those interested in bodybuilding, it's essential to prioritize both strength training and proper nutrition. Building lean muscle mass not only enhances your physique but also boosts your metabolism, making it easier to maintain a healthy weight. Remember to celebrate your progress by setting achievable goals and tracking your improvements in strength and muscle definition.

Barre workouts, originally designed for dancers, have gained popularity among women seeking a graceful and toned physique. These workouts combine elements of ballet, Pilates, and yoga to sculpt long, lean muscles and improve flexibility. Celebrate your achievements in barre by mastering challenging movements or noticing improvements in your balance and posture.

No matter your fitness niche, it's crucial to prioritize self-care and listen to your body. Regular rest days, proper nutrition, and adequate sleep are essential for long-term success. By celebrating your achievements and maintaining a balanced approach to fitness, you can stay motivated, prevent burnout, and enjoy the journey towards a strong and sculpted body.

Remember, fitness is not just a destination but a lifelong journey. Celebrate your achievements, embrace new challenges, and continue to prioritize your health and well-being. Strong and sculpted, you are capable of achieving anything you set your mind to.

Chapter 8: Fitness Beyond the Gym: Incorporating Physical Activity into Everyday Life

Finding Opportunities for Physical Activity in Your Daily Routine

In today's fast-paced world, finding time for exercise can often seem like an insurmountable challenge. However, incorporating physical activity into your daily routine doesn't have to be a daunting task. With a little creativity and determination, you can find numerous opportunities throughout your day to get moving and stay active. This subchapter aims to provide women, whether they are fitness enthusiasts, high-intensity interval training (HIIT) enthusiasts, bodybuilders, or dancers seeking barre workouts, with practical tips to seamlessly integrate exercise into their daily lives.

1. Commuting Creatively: Instead of relying solely on your car or public transportation, consider walking, cycling, or rollerblading to your destination. Not only will this help you burn calories and improve cardiovascular health, but it will also save you money on transportation costs.

2. Deskercise: Take regular breaks from your desk job to stretch, perform squats, or do quick bursts of aerobic exercises. These mini-workouts can help combat the negative effects of prolonged sitting and improve your overall fitness level.

3. Family Fitness: Involve your loved ones in physical activities, such as hiking, biking, or playing sports. This not only promotes a healthy lifestyle for everyone but also strengthens family bonds.

4. Lunchtime Workouts: Utilize your lunch break to squeeze in a quick workout. Whether it's a HIIT session, a bodybuilding routine, or a barre workout, even a 30-minute exercise session can have significant benefits for your physical and mental well-being.

5. Household Chores: Transform mundane household chores into calorie-burning opportunities. Vacuuming, mopping, gardening, or even doing laundry can be turned into effective workouts by adding extra movements and intensity.

6. Active Socializing: Instead of meeting friends for coffee or dinner, choose activities that involve physical movement. Go for a hike, try an indoor rock climbing session, or take a dance class together. It's a great way to catch up while staying active.

7. Mindful Technology Use: Minimize sedentary screen time by incorporating physical activity into your tech routine. Use exercise apps, follow online workout videos, or invest in a standing desk to stay active while working or watching TV.

Remember, incorporating physical activity into your daily routine is not about finding huge blocks of time but rather making small, consistent efforts throughout the day. By embracing these opportunities, you'll not only improve your fitness level but also experience increased energy, enhanced mood, and overall better health. So start small, stay consistent, and watch as the benefits of an active lifestyle unfold before your eyes.

Making Exercise a Family Affair

In today's fast-paced world, it can be challenging for women to find time for themselves and prioritize their fitness goals. However, by turning exercise into a family affair, you can not only achieve your fitness goals but also create a strong bond with your loved ones. In this subchapter, we will explore the benefits of making exercise a family activity and how you can involve your family members in your fitness journey.

Fitness is not just for individuals; it can be a fun and enjoyable experience for the whole family. By getting everyone involved, you not only set a positive example for your children but also create an environment that promotes health and well-being. Whether it's going for a family walk, playing sports together, or engaging in group workouts, there are numerous ways to make exercise a part of your family's routine.

One popular trend in the fitness world is high-intensity interval training (HIIT), which is known for its effectiveness in burning calories and getting results in a short amount of time. HIIT workouts are perfect for families as they require little to no equipment and can be done in the comfort of your own home. You can create a circuit-style workout that includes exercises suitable for all fitness levels, allowing everyone to participate and feel accomplished.

Bodybuilding for women is another niche that can be adapted for a family setting. While weightlifting may seem intimidating, it is an excellent way to build strength and sculpt your body. By incorporating bodybuilding exercises into your family workouts, you can teach your children about the importance of strength training and dispel the myth that it is only for men.

For those with a passion for dance, barre workouts can be a fantastic option. Barre workouts combine elements of ballet, Pilates, and yoga to create a unique and challenging exercise experience. Not only will you improve your flexibility and posture, but you can also involve your family members in these graceful and fun workouts. Children can benefit from the coordination and balance exercises, while adults can enjoy the toning and sculpting effects.

Remember, the key to making exercise a family affair is to make it enjoyable and inclusive. Find activities that everyone can participate in and accommodate different fitness levels. By prioritizing your family's health and well-being, you create a positive environment that fosters a love for fitness and encourages everyone to lead an active lifestyle.

In conclusion, by making exercise a family affair, you not only achieve your fitness goals but also create lasting memories and stronger bonds with your loved ones. Whether you choose high-intensity interval training, bodybuilding, or barre workouts, involve your family members in the process and prioritize their health. Together, you can embark on a fitness journey that will benefit everyone involved.

Incorporating Fitness into Social Gatherings and Events

As women, we are always looking for ways to stay fit and healthy while still enjoying our social lives. The good news is that you don't have to choose between fitness and fun! In this subchapter, we will explore the exciting world of incorporating fitness into social gatherings and events. From high-intensity interval training (HIIT) to bodybuilding for women and barre workouts for dancers, there are numerous ways to stay active while having a great time with friends.

One popular trend in fitness is HIIT, a form of exercise that combines short bursts of intense activity with rest periods. Imagine hosting a fitness-themed party where you and your friends engage in fast-paced HIIT workouts together. Not only will you get a great sweat session, but you'll also bond with your friends through the shared experience of pushing yourselves to the limit. It's a win-win situation!

For those looking to build strength and sculpt their bodies, bodybuilding for women is a fantastic option. You can organize a bodybuilding competition among your friends, complete with judges, trophies, and even a red carpet. This event will not only motivate you to reach your fitness goals but also serve as a celebration of your hard work and dedication.

If you have a passion for dance, barre workouts are an excellent choice. Why not organize a barre dance party where you and your friends can learn new moves while getting a full-body workout? You can hire a professional instructor to guide you through the session, or simply follow along with online tutorials. The beauty of this event is that it combines fitness with the joy of dance, allowing you to express yourself while toning your muscles.

Incorporating fitness into social gatherings and events not only keeps you active but also adds a unique and exciting element to your social life. By choosing activities that align with your interests, such as HIIT, bodybuilding, or barre workouts, you can combine your passion for fitness with the pleasure of spending time with friends. So why not host your next gathering with a fitness twist? Your body and mind will thank you for it!

Remember, staying fit doesn't mean sacrificing fun and socializing. With the right mindset and creative ideas, you can transform any gathering into a fitness-centered event that leaves you feeling energized and fulfilled. So grab your friends, lace up your sneakers, and get ready to have the time of your life while working towards your fitness goals!

Embracing an Active Lifestyle for Lifelong Health and Wellness

In today's fast-paced world, it's more important than ever for women to prioritize their health and wellness. Leading a sedentary lifestyle can have detrimental effects on our physical and mental well-being. That's why it's crucial for women to embrace an active lifestyle that promotes lifelong health and wellness. In this subchapter, we will explore various fitness options such as high-intensity interval training (HIIT), bodybuilding for women, and barre workouts for dancers, all of which can help women achieve their fitness goals and lead a healthier life.

High-intensity interval training (HIIT) has gained immense popularity in recent years, and for good reason. This form of exercise involves short bursts of intense activity followed by brief recovery periods. HIIT workouts are known to boost metabolism, burn calories, and improve cardiovascular health. Whether you're a beginner or a seasoned fitness enthusiast, HIIT provides a challenging yet rewarding workout that can be tailored to individual fitness levels.

Bodybuilding is often associated with men, but it's equally beneficial for women. Contrary to popular belief, bodybuilding for women doesn't mean bulking up but rather building lean muscle mass and sculpting a strong physique. Strength training not only helps improve bone density, but it also enhances overall body composition, boosts metabolism, and promotes better posture. With the right guidance and training programs, women can achieve a toned and sculpted physique that exudes confidence.

For those with a passion for dance or simply looking for a fun and effective workout, barre workouts for dancers are an excellent choice. Inspired by ballet, barre workouts combine elements of dance, Pilates, and strength training to create a unique fitness experience. These workouts focus on toning and strengthening muscles, improving flexibility, and enhancing posture. Barre workouts are low-impact, making them suitable for women of all fitness levels while still delivering impressive results.

No matter which fitness niche you choose to explore, the key is to find an activity that you enjoy and can stick to in the long term. Embracing an active lifestyle is not just about achieving short-term fitness goals but rather about making positive changes that can positively impact your overall health and well-being for a lifetime. So, lace up your sneakers, grab your workout gear, and embark on a journey of self-discovery, strength, and lifelong health and wellness. Your body and mind will thank you.